I0505064

More than Medicine: What They Don't Teach You in Medical, MA, Nursing or PA School

*Practical **Tips** to improve your bedside manner, manage staff & patients, & set you apart from other healthcare providers!*

Printed in the United States of America

ISBN: 978-1508979579

Acknowledgements & Dedication

First, I thank God for giving me the experiences and insights needed to create this book.

This book is dedicated to my loving and supportive parents and my grandma. Thank you for always being moral compasses for me to emulate.

To my mother, who also handled the editing of this work, I could not have done it without you.

I would also like to dedicate this book to my amazing husband, Laraun, who has been and continues to be my best friend and my #1 fan. Thank you!

Table of Contents

Preface: Why?

"You win with people."

-Woody Hayes

That statement pretty much sums up the many reasons why I wrote this book. As a young and eager student doctor, I was made acutely aware of the lack of inter-personal skills and bedside manner that exists in the medical field. When talking with patients and their family members I was told of so many horror stories of negative experiences they had with doctors, nurses, staff and paraprofessionals. In their time of pain and illness, the medical personnel who should be providing care, solace and compassion were the ones who sometimes added to their despair.

Similarly, as I made my way through residency training and entered into corporate America, I was again hit with the realization that there was a need for medically related personal skills training- for direct patient care staff as well as administrative staff.

There are two common questions that are always at the forefront of healthcare:

1. How does a practice hire *and* keep good, hard-working STAFF?
2. How can healthcare providers see patients quickly while still providing excellent medical care?

Both of these questions ultimately affect the bottom line – *revenue.* As time went on, I began searching for books and material to help not only myself, but others. When I could not find such information, I decided to compile tips that I use daily, in the hope that the information will help us all to be more effective and efficient healthcare providers.

With all the changes in healthcare costs and the increase in patients' desire to be healthier and more in control of their health, it is imperative for healthcare providers to simply be the best. Patients have choices. If they are not pleased with you or your staff/customer service they will simply search online for a different provider. Gone are the days when patients kept a provider even if they were unhappy with the services rendered.

There are numerous websites and blogs that rate, grade and give candid patient feedback. People are talking about their experiences face-to-face and on social media. The world-wide-web has made it possible for the *world* to have access to *your* patient care profile; good or bad. Remember, anything on the internet is potentially permanent. There is a footprint of every posting and picture.

Additionally there are websites that are geared toward giving patients just enough information to 'self-diagnose'; whether their diagnoses are correct or not. So what does this mean for you, as a healthcare provider? You have to provide complete, directed excellent services to your patients, without exception. Bad news travels fast. Unfortunately we are human and thus flawed and there are limitations, such as time, which play a factor. Our goal is to please every patient, sadly that is not always possible.

So how can you provide an excellent patient experience while being efficient? The ways may surprise you in their simplicity. Though simple, the ways are not always easily executable amidst full patient schedules, constant phone calls, charting, surgeries, patient /family consultations, et cetera.

The good part is that you have already taken the first step which is making the *decision* to be excellent and efficient. To be set apart from the thousands of other healthcare professionals by honing your inter personal skills and not just your didactic knowledge. After all, the world-wide-web has given people reason to believe that they can diagnose and treat themselves without the face-to-face care provided by doctors, nurses and paraprofessionals. You know differently. Your expertise is priceless; though one look at the student loan debt for doctors and other medical professionals may be able to give a price tag!

Finally, before you get started, I want to inform you that this book is not written using "their" and "them" as singular pronouns but instead uses the masculine pronouns "he" "his" and "him" to include both male and female.

*I once spoke with a patient
who was extremely upset
because her previous doctor
was trying to explain her
condition and treatment
options with an analogy that
she did not understand-
roofing. She was an English
teacher, very well educated,
but knew nothing about
roofing. Even after explaining
that she did not understand
the point the doctor was
making, he continued on with
the analogy for the entire
visit. She left frustrated,
confused and without any
clear understanding of her
pathology, etiology or reasons
for treatment.*

Chapter 1:

Getting Started

This book is not going to give you gross anatomy tips, biochemistry memorization acronyms or outline the ways to ace standardized tests. That part you have to do on your own. Don't despair though; most celebrated geniuses don't even have a college degree. You will be fine. What you will get from this book are various means that I employ when dealing with my patients, co-workers, staff and colleagues. These tips will enable you to serve your patients better and have a more positive work environment.

The saying goes that if you want to keep a secret, put it in a book! You are the smart one, you bought this book and have invested in yourself and your success. Good job! Let's get started.

Initial Cues

When first entering the room, take a moment to look around.

- Is the patient reading a book or magazine?

- Is he playing on his phone?
- Is he sitting with his eyes closed or is he peering at the door with eyes wide open like a deer in headlights?
- Does the patient quickly greet you or is he more reserved and waiting for you to speak?
- When you extend your hand or offer a verbal salutation, is he rapid with his verbal and non-verbal response, or more paced and deliberate?
- Are his hands folded across his chest, resting on his lap or is he fidgeting and restless?
- Does he have a list of questions or articles printed out with highlighting and personal notes?

The answers to these questions will set the tone for how you will meet your patient's needs most comfortably and effectively.

In order to allow time to assess the verbal and non-verbal cues, be sure to greet the patient and give good eye-to-eye contact and ask a general basic question: "Hello Mr. / Mrs. Smith, how are you today?" Then actually *LISTEN AND WAIT* for a response. During that time survey the room and watch your patient's posture.

The following are some verbal and non-verbal cues, with a corresponding deduction:

Table 1.

PATIENT/ENVIRONMENT CUES	SAFE ASSUMPTION/DEDUCTION	CAREGIVER'S ACTION
Sitting with arms folded, legs crossed, inexpressive facial and voice gestures	Closed stance	Ask open-ended questions to get good history
Twitching extremity, biting lip, brow sweating	Nervous about appointment; severe pain/symptoms	Reassure and instill confidence; verbalize that pain/symptom relief is top priority
Patient with children/young child	Time is limited and there will be distractions	Verbalize intent to be mindful of time; Include child in directed assistance*
List of questions, printed articles and handwritten notes	Fact-oriented, appreciates direct answers and reading material	Provide statistics, patient education material
Very energetic, bubbly and carefree with gestures	Easy going, appreciates light conversation	Use layman's terms vs medical terms

*Ask the child for help by letting him hold safe, simple equipment, opening drawers, or holding the patient's hand for support. Ask the child if he has questions. These are all ways to keep a child entertained so he will be less of a distraction, while building a rapport with your patient. Those who are with patients in an intimate setting such as an examination room, are dearly valued by the patient.

Get Connected

If you have not already, you will realize that time is money, literally. So, not only do you have to be an exceptional practitioner, you also have to be efficient and effective. As much as you would like to spend an hour with every patient, it is not possible, nor should it be expected of you. Still, patients do expect that of you; after all, some have taken time off from work to see you. Their time is valuable also, and they deserve your undivided attention.

What's in a Name?

Have you ever noticed that when you are speaking with customer service representatives they are *constantly* saying your name? At times, I admit it is annoying. Their goal though is to create a sense of relationship and rapport with you, quickly. A few years ago my husband and I had the pleasure of staying at the Ritz Carlton Hotel in Montego Bay, Jamaica. I will never forget the excellent customer service and attention to detail the staff displayed. The door man, the random gardener tending to the rose bushes, and the bartender knew our names and when we walked by them in the hall or passed them by the pool, they said "Hello Mr. & Mrs. Josey!" It was literally shocking! I am sure they must have all had some sort of earpiece or other communication device, for I surely do not know how every staff member knew us by name! It made us feel welcomed and comfortable. When you enter a room, be sure to greet your patient and the patient's companions. Whether you say your patient's first name or surname, this will create a connection and demonstrate your genuine interest in your patient. In addition, by saying your patient's name, it can help prevent patient mix-ups. Trust me, when things get hectic and you have multiple rooms with waiting patients, the last thing you want to do is begin to treat and discuss a diagnosis with the wrong patient!

Sympathy & Compassion

I have heard of too many horror stories where healthcare professionals relay bad news and new diagnoses without any sympathy or an attempt at empathy for the patient. Patients are left feeling hurt, sad, confused and upset. Depending on your field, even fatal prognoses may become common. It is important that you do not become callus to the patients sitting in your chair. For you, it may be a diagnosis that you have discussed with patients a thousand times over; but for the patient, it is a life altering moment.   Always, even when busy and stressed, remain compassionate.

To nurses, medical assistants, physician assistants as well as other paraprofessionals (front desk staff included), I must reiterate that sympathy and empathy are *not* just for the physicians. Quite the opposite. After years of practicing as a doctor, I realize that patients and family members will tell paraprofessionals certain details of their concerns and patient history, which they often omit when talking to

> A 65-year-old male patient with sleep apnea told the nurse, but not the doctor, he was using his cousin's Vicodin ES medication to ease his pain. This is a recipe for disaster and may lead to death. This information is a 'must know' so that the patient can be educated about the possible risk of death from his actions.

the doctor. That being said, your role in appropriately consoling and providing empathy and sympathy is large. In addition, when your patient shares information with you, but does not share it with the physician, it is your duty to tell the physician what the patient said.

Laughter

Laughter is a universal ice breaker. Your job is not to be a comedian, but making your patient smile puts everyone at ease. As a podiatrist, I like to say things like, 'go ahead and take both of your shoes off, we are having a two for one special today', or 'sorry, my x-ray vision is not working today, you will have to take your shoes off for me to do your exam.' These little statements help to ease tension and usually crack the expected monotony of a medical visit.

Family Members

If patients bring a friend or family member with them that is usually an indication that they value said person or that person is very active in their medical care. I have found that involving friends and family in the patient's medical history as well as treatment plan can be helpful, at times. It is known in the medical community that patients remember very little of what is actually said to them, by their healthcare provider. Having another set of ears is always helpful for patients. Plus, patients tend to omit important information during their history, and having someone else there to provide details is very helpful.

Additionally, developing a rapport with family members and friends is extremely important when you consider that they are a warm market for new business. Asking questions and directing statements toward present friends and family are quick and easy ways to develop a relationship. All it takes is including them in the conversation. I have found that usually I can generate one or more new patients per week, solely from patient family and friends being in the room. This, coupled with other marketing strategies can really increase your business! Taking the extra minute to answer the friend's 'so, doc what should I do about…?' question is a minute well spent.

Personalize the Visit

Little gestures like saying happy birthday or happy belated birthday can positively influence your patient's experience. Commonly, patients complain that they feel like a mere chart number or a diagnosis. Your goal should be to personalize the patient visit. When formalizing the treatment plan or goals be sure to include religious values, cultural norms, hobbies, et cetera. If you know that your patient is an avid golfer, make reference to that when speaking of getting more exercise. If your patient has grandchildren, encourage him to make better health choices so he can live long enough to enjoy his grandchildren. Use your patient's hobbies to make appropriate analogies and help him understand his diagnosis or to make your point. For some healthcare providers, they are able to easily remember details about their patients. For others, making notes for themselves is a fool proof way to personalize the visit. I have heard a quote that says: 'always trust a dull pencil over a sharp mind'. So, if you need to make notes on the chart, do so!

Take a moment to ask about a recent vacation or inquire about the health of a family member that you know is ill. You will soon find that patients equate good inter-personal skills with superior care. Hence the importance of bedside manner. In short, you want to let people know that your concern is for *them entirely,* not only their diagnoses. You want to convey that you care about them, beyond the confines of the office, including their quality of life. Reminding your patients that a consequence of poorly controlled diabetes can lead to impotence and vision loss, usually gets their attention, and it becomes more of a quality of life concern for them vs. just blood glucose numbers and HbA1c's.

Eye Contact
Never trust someone who does not look you in the eye when he is talking to you. We have all heard that and probably feel that way too. When dealing

with patients, it is important to build a rapport of trust. Maintaining eye contact is a vital part of that rapport. In addition, speaking deliberately and well-paced is important to help give the patient time to process what you are saying. Remember, for you, the information is common knowledge and you will probably say it a hundred times in a week; for your patient, it is new information, so he needs time to understand what you are saying and formulate questions, accordingly. With the requirement of electronic medical records, we are forced to spend hours looking on the computer or tablet screen. Be mindful of this and be sure to use your eyes to communicate with your patient. Eye contact speaks volumes about your character and it translates into a genuine relation to your patient.

Share

Share about yourself! Minor information, makes people feel like they know you and it makes the visit more personal. Everyone wants to feel as though they have a connection with their hairdresser/barber, their local bank teller, and especially their healthcare provider. A minute of small talk goes a long way, in patient perception. Depending on the situation I will do one of two approaches:

1. If time permits, I will pause the physical exam, and make small talk. I will ask about his family, weekend plans, or a book I notice he is reading, et cetera. During that time you want to show that you are actively listening to your patient: making eye contact, asking questions, and giving comments are all important. If possible, I will indicate some minor detail about my life. I have found that patients like it when they know you are a real person, more than just an amazing doctor! Also, amidst a busy day, having a patient ask about how *my* son is doing, really brightens my day. Every parent wants to brag!

2. If time is limited, I will make small talk *while* I am conducting the physical exam. Breaking throughout to get the patient's feedback while palpating and such, of course.

The overall patient perception will be that you have spent more time with the patient then you actually have. Even if you are in a rush, your patient will not feel slighted, because the visit had *personal substance* and not just a medical focus.

Touch

Too often, from my patients, I have heard that I have been the first doctor to actually do a tactile exam

on them. They have complained that most of their
healthcare providers simply sit at the computer
screen asking questions and typing. Never looking at
them, or even examining the areas of concern.
Diabetics sit in my office and say that no one has ever
looked at their feet before. That is ludicrous. Not only
is it poor patient care to omit tactile examinations, but
it also negatively impacts the patient's perception
during the visit. Some patients have even told me that
they sense their healthcare providers are scornful of
them. That is definitely the last thing you want a
patient to sense.

True, we do come across patients who could
use a lesson in personal hygiene, or who have
unpleasant presentations, but that is the nature of our
job. It comes with the territory, and gloves and masks
are meant to be used.

Before leaving the exam room, sometimes
providing a comforting touch on the shoulder can
make the world of a difference. There are times when
you will simply be seeing a patient as a follow up to
see how he is responding to a certain medication or
treatment plan. There may be no logical reason to do
another physical exam.   Still remember the
importance of non-verbal communication. Tactile
communication can add value to your patient's

perception of an otherwise basic patient encounter, giving assurance that it was not a waste of time to come back for a mere 'follow-up'.

Summarize

Once you have come to the end of your examination and treatment plan, give the patient a quick recap of his diagnoses and treatment options. Have the patient repeat what you said, back to you, if you are concerned that he does not understand. A large part of patient compliance is comprehension.

Educational Material

Patients are more prone to be compliant and follow the treatment plan if they have material to review when they leave the office. Having a few brochures to give to your patients is a great way to connect with them, even after they leave. Also, be sure to add your office contact information for easy access. I believe that patients, in normal circumstances recall about 50-60% of the information given to them, verbally.

Food for Thought

When dealing with new patients or return patients you should always be thinking as a healthcare provider, as well as a salesman. Yes, you are in the sales business. Every person is as a matter of fact.

You are the CEO and manager of YOU, Inc. If your patient likes you, he will refer his family and friends to you. If he likes you, he will be more willing to pay the copay. If your patient likes you, he will be more apt to follow your advice and treatment regimen. People do business with people they like. Contrary to what we have been lead to believe, medicine is indeed a business. A business thrives on referrals and new customers. As a doctor, medical assistant, nurse, or physician assistant you will know that you are truly connecting with your patients, when you begin to see their family members and friends schedule appointments with you.

Chapter 2: The Upset Patient

The Patient who is upset with a different provider

Very early in my medical career I realized that there were patients that I would not be able to please. Even if I relieved them of their ailment and pain, and even if I bent over backwards trying to accommodate their needs; some people are just not happy, and will not be happy with you, or any other provider, for that matter. Others are truly in pain and their pain is not only physically taxing but emotionally impacting their quality of life. It is our duty to be the best provider we can, for those patients. Not lending ourselves to speaking ill of our colleagues, especially since we are not able to totally know the circumstances surrounding the patient's history and treatment course with other providers.

With ambulance chasing lawyers and patients that are malingering, it is hard at times to decipher who are actually telling the truth and do have legitimate grounds to be upset. Still, as a healthcare provider, I think that the less I get involved with legal complaints, the better. Just agreeing with a patient's sentiments or frustrations when he is venting can put you in a position where you are viewed as agreeing that the patient has valid complaints against another provider. Frank agreement should be avoided when possible. Personally, I do not want to get involved in situations like those, unless it is an absolute must. If you practice long enough, you will have an irate patient...do not forget the golden rule-do unto others as you would have them do unto you.

When the patient has valid points of concern or complaint, and you would surely otherwise say that, it is not a good practice to have a lengthy conversation with the patient about his grievance with another provider. It gives the patient ammunition that can truly be hurtful to your colleague. However, there are cases of gross negligence or wrong doing that are hard to overlook. I usually take the following approaches:

Redirect the negative focus by doing the following:

1. Acknowledge (not agree with) their emotions, *briefly.* The less you ask about their issues with the other provider, the less involved you will become, thus preventing you from being caught in an awkward situation.
2. Speak highly of your colleague, if you do have a direct knowledge of him/her. We are all in the medical field together, and thus we are at the

same risk for having a disgruntled patient. If you do not know the provider in question, no need to lie. Assure your patient that there are many ways to manage and treat his condition, and each provider has treatment plans that he has found to work better than others, for his practice.

(It is very important not to down play your patients' emotions or

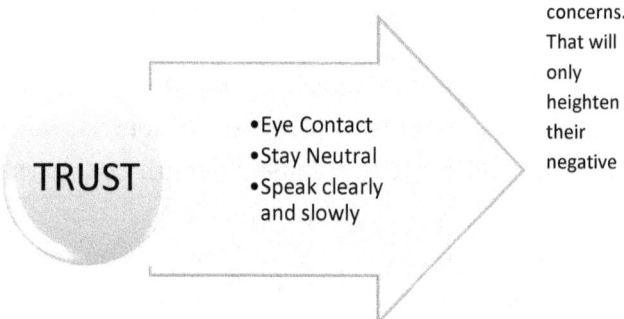

concerns. That will only heighten their negative

•Eye Contact
•Stay Neutral
•Speak clearly and slowly

TRUST

disposition. Instead, be direct in your acknowledgement of their issues and affirm that you will do your best to help them. Eye contact is extremely important. Also do not rush through this step, speak deliberately and clearly. People only care about what you are saying, when they know you care).

3. Then, without leaving too much time for rebuttals, begin to focus on their concern today and not what happened with the other provider. Remember he who asks the questions, controls the conversation. Immediately start asking medical history questions. Duration of symptoms, type of symptoms, treatments tried, et cetera. Your

goal is to get the focus towards their medical issue. At times, patients will begin again to bring in non-medical information, and information that is meant to discredit the other provider. Just repeat steps 1-3.

The Patient who is upset with you

Patients will get mad or upset with you. Maybe you are running behind and they are mad because they had to wait, maybe you did not give them pain medication/narcotics, or perhaps they did not get improvement of their symptoms with the treatment you rendered. Regardless of the reason, it is never a pleasant experience when you have an irate patient.

Doctors have been wearing white coats for over 100 years. Historically, it was used to distinguish quacksalvers and medieval medicine from modern scientific medicine. In the 1800s the white coat was donned as a symbol of cleanliness. Others use white coats for protection in laboratory settings. Currently white coats are worn by medical practitioners (mostly doctors) in an attempt to have an easily recognized symbol of scientific representation.

I have noticed that whereas most patients will be very vocal about their ill feelings with my staff (nurses, medical assistants, front desk personnel), they are usually less caustic when I enter the room.

White coat syndrome is a real effect for some patients. I have had patients with normal blood pressure testing before I enter the room, have increased heart rate and elevated blood pressure once I enter the room. Then, following the completion of the visit, their vitals return to normal range.

There is definitely a psychosomatic correlation between such instances, which is not relevant to the scope of this book. All you need know is that your white coat does have its drawbacks and perks; but such perks should not be abused and when the one donning the white coat is in error it is best to address it face on. People respect candor and are more apt to move on from a negative experience if they know that their concerns have been heard and addressed.

The white coat usually brings about a sense of respect for the one wearing it. Patients are *usually* less confrontational when the doctor (or anyone with a white coat) comes in. That being said, if you are aware that you patient is not happy with you or your staff, be sure to address his concern immediately and with sincerity. Your goal is to de-escalate the upset patient and swiftly change the course of his emotions from negative to positive.

Remember, it can take months to get a patient in the door, and just one second to lose him forever; not to mention the referral pool that patients bring with them. Some healthcare professionals do not really focus on the importance of customer service. It is vital, in order to set yourself apart from the rest. There are thousands of eager, bright, intelligent men and women matriculating in medicals schools all over the United States, alone.   At the time this work was penned, the Association of American Medical Colleges reported 20,000 first time enrollees and almost 50,000 total applicants. That is not including nursing, medical and physician assistants or specialty services such as audiology, dentistry, optometry, podiatry, physical medicine, et cetera. Your goal is to be distinguished and unique, not only in your skills and patient care but also in your customer service approach.

I have found the following ways to de-escalate the irate patient very helpful:

1. Acknowledge his emotion – anger, frustration, fear, anxiety. Unless you are in psychology/mental health, you do not need to delve into the depths of his emotions, but acknowledging his feelings is important. People want to be heard.

2. Empathize – we have all been upset before, so put yourself in your patient's shoes. Instead of being callus or indifferent, think of a personal incident where you too, felt the way your patient feels. Think of how you would have liked your situation to be handled. Then, work to give your patient the treatment you would have wanted. The golden rule applies: Do unto others as you would have them do unto you.

3. The customer is always right (unless ethically he is wrong) – do not argue with patients. If you are running behind, explain your reason and keep it moving. If your staff was less than stellar, let your patient know you will investigate and handle the situation. If your patient is still symptomatic, professionally exude confidence and concern, and reassure him that it is your goal for him to get better. Bottom line is, keep it moving. You can do more damage than good by trying to tell a patient how he should feel.

4. Repeatedly redirect the conversation. Your patient may try to harp on their anger and frustration. Your goal is to always bring it back to the issue at hand – your patient's medical care.

The Drug Seeking Patient

Tip #3 brings me to a very important point. People will be people and sometimes you will encounter patients who are dishonest, pill seeking, malingering, et cetera. They too deserve respect and excellent care. That being said, it is not in your best interest to cave to the unethical requests of patients.

I have seen it all too often that good healthcare providers get bullied into unethical situations by their patients. Our Hippocratic Oath requires us to diagnose and treat patients, but that does not mean cower to them.

If you suspect a patient of malingering or pill seeking, do your research. Most of the time you are not the first provider he has tried to take advantage of. Here are a few ways to research your patient's history:

- Call his pharmacy (and local pharmacies) to see how many narcotic prescriptions he has active.
- Contact his primary care doctor to see if he has any other conditions he is not telling you about (such as mental health related issues or history of substance abuse).

- Look at his allergy list. If he has listed allergies to multiple over-the-counter pain medications or standard narcotics (ibuprofen, naproxen, acetaminophen, hydrocodone, and tramadol) that is reason to be curious but not judgmental. Ask him the nature of his allergy; some 'allergies' are actually side effects of the pain medications. For example, constipation or nausea with narcotics.

> *TIP: Do an internet search or ask your local pharmacist to see if your state has a prescription drug monitoring program that allows you to look at a patient's prescription medication history.*

- Talk to the patient, directly. Let him know that your goal is to get him better, not simply mask his symptoms. Using your judgment, you can get a good idea if someone is being genuine or not.
- Be firm. If you get the impression that he is drug-seeking as soon as you can, inform him that you will not be dispensing or prescribing any such medications. Get that option off of the table. Then move on in the visit.

Follow your first instinct. You do not want to become someone's 'drug doctor'. Such an infamous moniker travels fast in pill-seeking circles and you will find yourself inundated with patients who do not actually want to get better, they just want a diagnosis and pills.

If you are not comfortable prescribing a medication, do not do it. The moment you open that portal of supply, it will be very hard to close it - even if your intentions are good.

If you feel threatened or in danger from a malingering patient, the first step is NOT to be alone with the patient in the examination room.   Always bring another staff member in, both for security and to act as a witness.

In addition, your medical record charting should reflect that you did not give nor order any such medication. Some patients will wait until you leave the room to ask your staff to place medication orders, or even call back later to ask if staff can place medication orders, on your behalf. They realize that clinicians are very busy and that some staff members do have authority to call in medications. If your staff is well trained, they will either contact you to find out if they can place the prescription, or they will look in your notes to see if any mention was made of prescriptions. Either way, you always want to have a record of your encounter with the patient, so as to help prevent making a mistake of filling a prescription in error. I like to have alternative treatment plans for those who I suspect are malingering. With the topical compound medication options increasing, I tend to use those instead. Research other treatment options for your patients that are actually beneficial to them, without compromising your integrity. Consider physical therapy or dietary supplements. When possible, you should add value to the appointment, even if you are suspicious of a malingering patient. It may mean that he/she needs a consultation for pain management or mental health screening. Try not to dismiss a patient because of his flaws. As healthcare providers, it is our duty to care for the *entire* individual, even if it means leaving the comfort zone of our field and getting our patient the help he needs.

Once you have assessed your initial cues, dealt with the irate patient, and ruled out malingering, it is now time to work your medical magic! Your goal is to give the patient peace of mind. Even if you are not totally sure what his diagnosis is, or what the best treatment plan is for him. The key is honesty. I call it intellectual honesty and realistic improvement measures.

The Patient Who Refuses to Comply

Even though patients take time out of their day to come and sit in your waiting room, fill out your office's many forms and pay their copays that does not mean that they are actually going to do as you instruct. Shocking, but true. It can be very frustrating when dealing with a refusing patient. Usually, they do not get better, and they blame you for that. I cannot stress it enough how important documentation is. If you have a patient who is noncompliant, you must enter that into his medical record. Your record should not reflect slander or defamation of character; instead it should relay facts, only. Be sure to clearly document your attempts to educate the patient on the possible risks and complications that can occur from his noncompliance. In our litigious society, a healthcare professional needs to think medically and legally. Hope for the best, prepare for the worst.

Chapter 3: Minority Matters: Biases in the Workplace & Exam Room

You remember the cliques in high school and middle school? What about the school bully or the loud, rude science partner, and the passive aggressive snob? Sad news, if you have not already figured it out, corporate America has the same group dynamics. Older age and higher echelon professional accomplishments do not correlate to maturity. In fact, at times I think the inverse is true.

Being a minority in medicine is something most of us will experience at some point, in some form. Gender, race, nationality, specialty, rank, longevity of employment, and experience are all criteria that can create majority and minority groups. Seeing that I have fit into all of the aforementioned groups at some point, I have experienced a fair share of biases.

Let me first start by letting it be known that my innate nature is not to see race, color, or gender.

Though I respect ranking, it does not truly affect me. Also, I realize that healthcare providers tend to start their careers at a young age, and with little real world experience.   Actually, I only really began to see how these factors affect professional settings when I moved back to the United States, after having lived in Jamaica, West Indies for a few years. In Jamaica the quality of the person's character is heavily weighted.

That being said, you can only imagine my disgust, frustration and frank sadness, when I had to deal with colleagues, patients, and superiors who openly expressed biases. Yes, I did say openly. The details of these egregious acts are not germane to the context of this work, however, I will say that the lessons I learned, definitely are.

First, I had to stop the urge to take it personally. This is not easy by any stretch of the imagination, because the actions of my offenders were definitely directed toward me. After all, I am usually the only black female surgeon in the room or group; no mistaking there. Still, I realize that if it were not me, it would be someone else as the target. That being said, I stopped making it about me, and more about their issues. By not taking it personally, you decrease the negative strength of the offense and you can handle it without being clouded by anger or pain.

Second, I have come up with a few witty statements that I routinely use to gently reprimand the offender, while providing him with information. When a patient questions my race, age or gender, my reply is: "Well, you do know that doctors now come in all different, colors, shapes, sizes, ages and genders!" This is said with a large, sincere smile, and looking them directly in the eyes. Nothing more needs to be said after that, anyone worth their weight in water, will get the picture and is usually quick to make amends.

Another option is to simply introduce yourself. Again, giving direct eye contact. When my peers ignore me or attempt to belittle me professionally, I speak up more and with more conviction and begin to ask them questions. Asking questions puts you back in control. That is if you care enough. The more experience I obtained, the less I cared. When you do good work, you will become well-known. The attitude of your peers will change. For those patients who express their concern about being treated by me (for whatever reason) I make it my goal, during that encounter, to be so very compelling in my evaluation and treatment plan that they will have a hard time maintaining their previous reservations.

I was listening to Dr. Ben Carson's *One Nation* audiobook, and he gave a great suggestion for how he dealt with such situations. He states that when he is mistaken for an orderly or other paraprofessional, he says something along the lines of, 'well I am sure that when the orderly arrives then they can definitely take the patient to their room; but I am Dr. Carson, so I will be performing the patient's surgery.' I think that is so clever! I wish I thought of that retort at times when I was prepping my room for surgery and the charge nurse reminded me to set up the fluoroscopy machine so that the doctor, (I), would not have any delays.

Bottom line is that the medical field is still very much a male, Anglo- Saxon dominated profession. For me that is quite alright, now. With more wisdom, and maturity, I welcome the looks of shock or confusion when patients see my name and title on my white coat, or better yet when they ask if the real doctor is coming in. I politely smile (using every ounce of self-control) and I inform them that I am the 'real doctor'. Then I make it my duty to give them the best, most professional care possible. In the end, they usually leave the office professing how impressed they are with the care they received.

See, when dealing with the biases and prejudices of others, it is always important to remember that you can be the person who changes their perspective for the better, or worse. Take that onus of responsibility seriously!

Finally, even with all of these tips and perspective changes, you will still have to deal with closed-minded people. It is inevitable. During residency,

"No one can make you feel inferior without your consent. " E-Roosevelt

I had an attending physician blatantly say that he did not like dealing with people with a Jamaican accent. WHAT?!?! Who says that? Such a rude, blanket statement! My accent, though less obvious now, is a part of who I am. In short, those with prejudices and biases are the ones with the issue- not you! Remember, most people who take issue with you, without even knowing you, have deeper problems that they need to resolve.

Chapter 4: The Flirt, the Know-It-All, the Talker, & the Unmotivated

The Flirting Patient

We have all dealt with the patient who thinks it is funny to make verbal and non-verbal advances. Here are a few ways I deal with the flirting patient:

1. Whenever possible try to have your wedding ring, or engagement ring on or in plain sight. On my surgery days, or when I am doing a procedure that requires me to remove my rings, I wear my wedding rings on a necklace around my neck. Now, some might say that the rings are less of a deterrent and might even heighten the interest of a flirting patient. Still, I think that it does speak volumes for a married person to have his ring on in public, because that shows that he is not hiding his married status.

2. If during the encounter/visit I pick up on verbal or non-verbal flirting, I will casually mention my husband, or the fact that I am married. Example: 'I totally understand what you are saying Mr. Doe, my husband complains

of the same pain after playing basketball.' Now, redirect the focus of the conversation. If you are not married, you can make the same statement about your significant other, or your brother, uncle, father, cousin, et cetera. When not speaking about a significant other or a spouse, the goal is to casually place the patient in the 'friends and family' zone. The same applies to female patients who are making inappropriate advances. Mention your mother, sister, aunt, or grandmother.

3. For those who are not married or in a serious relationship, it is a bit harder to professionally block the advances. When I was in such a position, I made sure to keep the verbal and non-verbal communications very pleasant but stoic. I did not do a lot of smiling, I used my 'doctor voice', and I did not easily laugh at jokes. Why not laugh you ask? Because men and women know that they are more likeable when they make someone laugh. Laughing heartily at a flirting patient's jokes, gives your admirer the courage and encouragement to continue. Most people get the idea when you continue to redirect the appointment to the medical business at hand.

4. In my field of podiatry, the physical examination does call for direct contact. I did not realize how many people would comment that my palpating their lower extremity for pain felt like a massage. At times, these sentiments would lead to inappropriate comments. Of course, that is never my intention. So, I ignore the comments completely, as though I did not even hear them say it.

5. When the advances are more direct, be equally direct. Inform the patient that the actions are not welcomed. Ask the patient to stop and then continue with the visit. If the patient does not stop the advances, leave the room and get someone to come back into the room with you. If all else fails and you are truly uncomfortable, ask the patient to leave. Your safety is important. Be sure to document the incident well. He who documents, usually wins. Speak with a legal professional or someone in human resources to find out the best way/place to document the incidents.

The Know-It-All Patient

The internet has become a major source of help and hindrance to the medical community. The internet is an invaluable resource from which to learn and share with others regarding medical skills and knowledge. The internet is also a great way for patients to become more enfranchised in their own health and medical care. By having access to symptoms and signs of diseases and illnesses, people are more apt to take an active role in their own healthcare. Nowadays, most patients come to the having already self-diagnosed, and after having tried multiple home remedies.

Therein lies the problem…not everything on the internet is true. Plus, there are many symptoms that are common to multiple diagnoses. In my experience, patients will recall some of what you say, but all of what the internet says.

So, dealing with patients who come in with a self-diagnosis and a treatment plan that they want for you to follow, is not only annoying, but it can be very counter-productive to their health success. When dealing with the 'know-it-all' patient, first realize that his knowledge, though sometimes correct, is from a lay person's perspective. At times, patients get confrontational if your diagnosis and treatment plan does not match their expectations.

First, do not argue with patients. It is not your goal to convince them that they are wrong.

Instead, the goal is to help them understand that you are right. Be patient and respectful of their perspective, but provide adequate information that will persuade them in your favor.

Being stern is also needed at times. Patients want to know when you are confident in their diagnoses and the ways to manage and treat them. If the patient is still not yielding or worse yet, states he will not cooperate with the treatment plan, then be frank but polite.

I remind my patients that they definitely have the choice of not heeding my recommendations, taking the medication, or making the lifestyle changes needed. However, I also inform them that they came to see a doctor for a reason. If they could have gotten rid of it on their own, then they would have. That usually gives them something to think about and makes them more apt to comply.

I have also found that some patients need to be reminded that you have spent years and years studying and learning about the various disease processes, body systems and ways to treat/manage ailments. When I am faced with a patient who shows signs that he too has been doing his 'homework' I choose to go into appropriate detail about his symptoms and diagnosis. Being sure to use medical terminology as though I am teaching a physiology class. No, the goal is not to be rude. The goal is to demonstrate to the patient that your knowledge is vast and that he is in good hands.

With holistic and homeopathic medicine gaining more popularity, I do like to have alternative methods of treatments available for those patients who qualify. I am by no means a homeopathic doctor. However, I do believe there is a place for holistic medicine, especially for those who are not keen on synthetic medications. When possible, research natural alternatives for pain, swelling, bruising, inflammation, nausea, et cetera.   This will really add to the value of your therapy for your patients.

Assert Yourself!
As healthcare professionals we assume that our patients are going to be compliant and attentive. We do not expect to get resistance against treatment plans nor do we expect to be told, by our patients, what they will and will not do. Though it does happen, the way in which we deal with this will surely set the tone for the entire medical relationship. When I am faced with patients who assert themselves negatively, I stay calm. There is no good that can

come from taking offense to their negativity. In fact, I not only stay calm, but the more negative they are, the more pleasant I try to be. Then, I firmly and politely explain that they have the option to take my medical advice and treatment plan, or they can ignore my advice. Then, I stop talking. That is right, I literally let the room become silent. I let the patient make the next move. More often than not, he will change his stance, because he did come to see you, the expert, after all. By giving the patient the option to move on with, or without your medical expertise, there is a fear of loss. The patient is now concerned that his layman's knowledge is not comparable to your expert opinion. Assert yourself!

The Talker

Time is money. Still, you should not cause or allow your patient to feel rushed during your encounter. In fact, most patient complaints are centered on the fact that the patient did not feel as though the healthcare provider devoted enough time to his needs. Before ending the patient encounter be sure to address the concerns, completely. Here are a few polite ways to end long-winded conversations without offending your patient.

1. Casually walk to the door and grab the door handle. Yes it works. It sends a subtle message that you are preparing to exit the room.

2. Ask a co-worker if your *next* patient is ready. Ask the question within earshot of your current patient. The goal is to give warning that you do have other patients waiting. If your patient is still not getting the hint, try being tactful and honest. Here is what I say, "I would love to talk to you all day but I have another patient waiting and I don't want them to wait because I am here running my mouth!" This makes your leaving more about being polite to the next patient and not being rude to your current patient.

3. Redirect the conversation by asking a question. Sometimes you will have to politely interrupt your patient to ask your question. The key is to be polite. I usually say, "Mr. Jones, I have a quick question." Then I proceed. This technique is actually helpful anytime you need to regain control of a conversation. When you ask your patient a question, it forces him to pay attention to you and thus you have control again. The question you ask should not be open-ended. Instead, ask a question that allows you to provide the last word. An

example would be inquiring if he understands the information you provided and his treatment course. If he answers 'yes', then the encounter has come to an end. Say your brief departure salutation and walk out. If he answers 'no' then you can summarize the information and then say your brief departure salutation and walk out. Win-win.

The Unmotivated Patient

At some time or another, you will deal with patients who are not actually motivated to get better. One might say, how can that be? They are coming to the office or clinic, seeking help. Well, I have found that at times, some people are more interested in talking or complaining about their ailments, than actually getting better. With that being said, your goal must still be to provide meaningful, caring treatment, even if they are not being compliant.

The first key is not to take it personally. Patients are regular people just like you and I. They can have bad days, stressful jobs, and financial issues too. So, just because they are not motivated to get better, does not mean that you are doing something wrong. So, before you get flustered and too annoyed, consider that other factors could be at play. Other factors can include: depression, financial limitations, lack of understanding, poor family/friend support, or even cultural barriers. The astute clinician will seek to find ways to influence and inspire the patient to be interested in getting better.

Here are some tips:

Table 2.

Problem	Solution
Depression or other mental health concern	If you suspect that mental health issues are at play, refer the patient to a therapist or counselor. If available, there may be programs in your local hospital's social work department.
Financial Limitations	Always strive to have cost conscious alternatives available. Consider using resources like pharmaceutical representatives and social workers, who have access to medication or device samples; plus they know of many programs available for financial hardship. Another option is to have supplies that are set aside for patients who cannot afford to get them otherwise.
Lack of Understanding	People tend to fear what they do not understand. If you suspect that lack of understanding is the culprit for poor compliance, take the time to educate your patient, in layman's terms, and have him repeat the information back to you.
Cultural Barriers	Be mindful that certain religions and cultures do not support modern medicine. Patients might be trying to use alternative vs. traditional medicine. If that is the case, it is important to carefully explain to them how your treatment plan will fit into their goals. Also, *if possible*, incorporate their ideas into your devised plan. Finally, attempt to *identify* and *dispel* any myths that may be hindrances.

Chapter 5: The Bad and the Ugly

Poor/Guarded Prognosis

The practice of medicine is truly just that - a practice. Though we are in the field of science, which is predicated on facts and logic, the human body is so very unique and intricate that not all ailments follow the rules of recovery, even with the best treatments.

Telling a patient bad news, or informing him of a poor or guarded prognosis is never easy. Unfortunately, it is a reality. The first few times you have to bear sad news, it may be a very humbling and emotional experience. With time, you will fall into your own comfort level and style of breaking sad news to patients and their families.

Here are a few tips I use when dealing with sad news:

1.   Maintain eye contact. Good eye contact lets your patients know you are being sincere and honest.

2. Speak in a calm, low tone. Your voice tone should express your sympathy or empathy, if appropriate.

3. Give your patient time to process what you are saying and ask if he has any questions. More than likely he will, but he may be in too much shock/sadness to formulate his thoughts. Urge him to write down any questions or concerns he has and bring them to his next appointment so you can discuss them together.

4. Sit or stand at eye level, never tower above them. If they are sitting, sit. If they are standing, then stand. This will create a more amicable atmosphere for communication.

5. Ask if he understands the news that you have given him? If he sits there with a blank stare, which may happen, repeat yourself.

6. Most importantly, if at all possible, do not deliver sad news/poor prognosis over the phone, via letter correspondence, email or any other means of communication that is not face-to-face. You do not know how people will take the news. You are not familiar with their support system, or lack thereof.

7. When possible and appropriate, have literature or other resources for information about their

diagnosis. I have found that an empowered patient is a calmer patient. Being empowered, even just with knowledge, allows people to process negative news better.

8. If family members or a friend is present, and the patient is in agreement, include the family members in the conversation. In my estimation, patients on a good day, without bad news, hear about 50-60% of what you say. So, having a second set of ears really helps. Plus, in the case of a very emotional response, having a family member or friend there to give physical consolation is far more appropriate.

Intellectual Honesty

Regarding intellectual honesty, this addresses the situations when you have a patient whom you are treating, but you are not totally sure what will be the best course of treatment, or if his diagnosis and treatment is outside of your scope of practice, or if you feel that his prognosis is guarded or poor. Patients appreciate honesty, even if it is uncertainty on your part. Nowadays, the internet allows everyone to quickly research and self-diagnose, and even cross check your diagnosis and treatment information. They may lose trust in your judgment because you were not honest about your limitations and their projected outcome.

Remember, you want to under promise and over deliver, when appropriate. Of course, if you are confident about their outcome, then by all means relay that confidence! However, if the converse is true, it will serve you better to be honest and forthright.

Here are a couple statements that I use often:

Mrs. Doe I like to be honest and upfront with you about our expectations for your outcome. Based on the nature of your presentation, while all of your pain/symptoms may not be resolved, if we improve them, we should consider that a win.

Mr. Doe your clinical exam is very complex and there are multiple factors that are contributing to your presentation. I want to get to the root cause of your symptoms, together. I like to have definitive diagnoses before I decide upon a full treatment plan. Let's get some more tests and work our way through the possible causes of your symptoms so we can get a concrete answer.

These statements convey confidence, a strategy, realistic goals, and give the patient a sense of team work. Patients often complain that they do not know why they are having certain tests done. By informing patients and explaining why they are having tests done, they are less likely to get upset or frustrated if the diagnosing process takes a few tries. Also, they will be more agreeable to fees and copays if they understand the reason for the tests. One of the easiest ways to upset a patient is to have him take a test or get lab work that he does not understand or did not consent to, then send him a huge bill.

Chapter 6: Staffing

Earning Respect from Staff/Co-Workers

The greatest challenge when dealing with staff and co-workers is gaining their respect. Most people give others the benefit of the doubt, initially. The struggle comes when you must deal with hierarchy and delegation of tasks.

As a young doctor and even during residency, I found that setting the tone for the professional relationship is vital, from the start. Think of your work relationship just as you would a marriage or a friendship. Do not do anything in the first six weeks, that you do not want to be the expectation for the remainder of the professional relationship. What does that mean? Well, if you do not want your co-workers to bring gossip and workplace rumors to you, do not involve yourself in such discussions from the start. If you do not want to be labeled as lazy, work hard from the first day, even if you think no one is watching.

When you are in the position to delegate, take note of who is willing and able to carry out certain tasks well. From day one, begin to recognize those who are sharp and eager. Take notice of persons who are coachable and hardworking. Begin to assign responsibility to such individuals and follow up regularly to see if the job was done, properly. By showing that you can and will delegate tasks, you are letting others know that you do have expectations of them. Respect will soon follow. Do not be afraid to give appropriate correction when you recognize areas in which your staff member needs to improve. By letting others know that you are actually paying attention and expecting them to do well, you are directly telling them that you do, in fact anticipate that they will give their best.

In turn, you too must be willing to give your best to your team and in your work. If you have expectations that you, yourself are not willing to meet, you set yourself up for ridicule and disrespect. The fastest way to lose the respect of your staff and co-workers is to follow the 'do as I say, but not as I do' philosophy.

Similarly, if you are already established in your workplace, and seeking to earn more respect from your co-workers/staff members, again, be sure you are displaying respect to them. You cannot expect from others, what you do not give to them. Then, begin to make small adjustments in your professional relationships. It will not be easy to create a different relationship dynamic, but it is possible. It will take time and effort on your part.

I find that edifying or uplifting others is a great way to begin a new foundation for even an old, established professional relationship. Remember, everyone likes to feel important and show how much knowledge they have about a certain topic or field of study. Acknowledging your co-worker's skills will make him more agreeable to doing tasks when asked and mutual respect will develop.

Take responsibility. When there is an issue, error or negative event, even if your role in the situation is minimal, take responsibility as a leader would. People respect leaders. Not to say that you become the scape goat for all errors in the office. No, that is not the goal. However, instead of being a part of the blame game, take ownership of aspects that you could have controlled, even if they are not directly related to your job description. What does that mean? Instead of pointing the finger at others when a patient is skipped, in error, and seen late, take ownership of what you could have done to avoid the error. Maybe you could have been more attentive to the schedule. Say so. People inherently equate responsibility with leadership and leadership with respect. Next, move on and give a *solution* to the problem.

Getting Staff On Board via the Pack Leader

The most direct way to get your staff on one accord is to identify and isolate the leader(s) of the staff/team. There is always one or more natural leaders in the pack. The pack leader is a person who can naturally persuade other staff members to do certain things or not do other things. The pack leader is the rate limiting step in the office productivity and he/she can set the tone for the entire office day; and even the expected culture and work environment on a daily basis. If you are in the position to, work closely with the leader of the pack. This individual is a key part of the office flow. If you want to introduce a new protocol, or get a point across, the pack leader can help get everyone else on board.

Dealing with Difficult Staff/Co-Workers

This section will only touch upon some highlight points when dealing with staff who are less than satisfactory. Of course, if you are the boss, well... the rules change a bit. If you too are an employee, then it becomes more of a challenge.

If you do not already know, you will soon find out that your staff members are the most important people in your practice. Treat them well. I will go into detail on building staff morale in a later chapter.

Your office staff is the first and last people who your patients see. First impressions matter, especially in medicine. So what should you do if you have a staff member who is not cutting it? Well, having a good employee manual is important. There should be consequences to poor work performance, and such consequences should be well outlined and performance errors should be documented.

Still, there are some employee issues that cannot be put into words or easily outlined in an employee manual. I once heard someone say that no one admits to poor work ethic on his resume.

Here are some scenarios and ways to handle them:

Table 3.

Employee Action	Your Response
Lack of respect for other staff members	In private, tell the staff member what you notice, and have actual instances where his actions were observed. Let him know that his actions are having a negative effect on the office atmosphere and that from now on you expect him to treat others with respect. Give him examples of ways to better handle adverse situations. Then, inform him that you will be monitoring his progress. Finally, set a date to review his progress.
Lack of respect for you	See above
Poor bedside manner	In private, tell the staff member what you notice, giving him tangible ways to improve his performance. Give positive reinforcement when appropriate!
Poor work performance	Record specific instances of poor performance and present them to your staff member, in private. Provide resources and trainings so he can improve. Give him a reasonable deadline by which to show improvement. Give positive reinforcement when appropriate and also record the performance issues and the ways in which he has been advised to correct them. Always refer to your employee handbook for termination guidelines.

Giving correction to staff

Here are some rules I use when approaching my staff and co-workers when I have to give correction or criticism.

1. **Sandwich method**: we have probably all heard of this tactic before. Basically saying a positive action that the person is doing or giving him a compliment, followed by the constructive criticism, and closed with another compliment or positive statement. The goal here is to soften the blow of the reproach, with sincerity. People are prone to get defensive when they are being corrected, so do not be alarmed if your co-worker gets defensive. Simply attempt to reassure him that you want the best for the company and for him.

2. **Privacy**: remember growing up as a child, and getting in trouble in front of the whole class? Yeah, it made matters worse, and the entire lesson was lost in the humiliation of the public moment. Instead, I recommend giving the correction in a private, one-on-one setting. Assure your staff that the conversation is private and that you have no intention of sharing the news with others. If he chooses to, that is his prerogative.

3. **Assurance**: most times when staff members are corrected, their initial concern is job security. When possible, do let them know that they have job security, unless that is not the case. If so, then being honest and forthright is best. I would not recommend having such a serious discussion without proper documentation and a managing co-worker for witness.

4. **Do Not Change**: after giving correction or criticism, it is often tense or awkward between you and the staff member. Attempt to maintain professionalism and avoid the tendency to act differently toward your staff member. Even if he acts differently toward you, just be the same way you were, and in no time, he should follow suit.

5. **Be Fair:** no one likes the teacher's pet...so if you correct one, correct all. People respect you more when they know that you are not showing curry favor with your constructive criticism. Of course you may have a more amicable relationship with certain co-workers, but that is not to interfere with your leadership or attitude toward your peers.

Connecting with Staff & Creating a Positive Work Environment

Compliments & Kudos:

Everyone wants to be appreciated and recognized. It is our human nature. Even if you are selfless, recognition matters. Hence, the best way to improve the morale of your staff and co-workers is to give them compliments/kudos. Everyone does something good or exceptional. Even the smallest of tasks, done well, can be a chance to boost someone's self-esteem. Confident people, who feel appreciated, are more productive and are more eager to do well. You get out, what you put in. That goes for your relationships with your staff and co-workers.

"People don't care how much you know, until they know how much you care." - Theodore Roosevelt

Most of us have had that boss or colleague who was negative, rude, tactless, obnoxious, who loved to nit-pick and find fault. Do not be that person. At times, you have to work and spend more time with your co-workers than your family, so strive to make it a pleasant experience.

"Thank you". Two simple words that have such an impact on your staff and even your co-workers. True, no one *has* to work with you or for you, and similarly they have a choice to do a good job versus a mediocre job.

Smile
Yes, simple truth. Smiles are contagious. Really not much that needs to be said here.

Listen
God gave us two ears, and one mouth. Active listening is vital to a positive work environment, and successful practice. When people feel heard, they feel valued. Even if you cannot change, or answer their question or concern at that moment, active listening can make the world of difference from a staff member feeling helpless and disenfranchised to wanting to be active in the solution to a concern/problem.

That leads me to another point. Delegating tasks to those who are capable, can add to team morale and give purpose to co-workers. If people develop a vested interest in the practice, they are prone to work harder, more diligently, and with more pride.

Care

Too often, we get self-absorbed and forget that we are a part of a team. Or, we get so bogged down with the day-to-day routine of the office, we neglect to *care* about staff and colleagues. Take a moment to pay attention to your staff and colleagues.   Ask about their family, their weekends, and their extra-curricular activities. Your goal is not to be 'nosey', instead, it is to create a real cordial relationship among your team.

Chapter 7: Awkward Situations & Time Saving Tips

How to Fire a Patient

Yes, you may have to do this at some point in your career. Remember those patients who are pill-seekers and malingerers? Sometimes you have to let them go, so that you can be effective for your other patients. Also, there

TIP: Always keep correspondence in patient's file. Do not discard.

TIP: Be sure to collect any monies or debt before discontinuation of services, as I am almost positive you will not get any money owed once they have received your letter.

are patients who have no intention of getting better, but instead just want to continue in their pain or frustration. They could have a mental health issue, and in such a case, would do well with a referral to a specialist.

Then, there are patients who are aggressive, rude and frankly ungrateful. I have a doctor friend who always reminds me that not all money, is good money! Such a basic but powerful truth. Just because a patient comes in with his copay, but disrespects you and your staff, does not mean that you have to continue to see him in the practice. One patient should not repeatedly spoil the entire schedule or day. Be smart about scheduling patients. The stress and upset that can come with problematic patients can ruin the flow of the rest of your day.

I am sure there are a few ways in which you can fire a patient, and you have to find the way that works best for you. Here are ideas:

Letter: Draft a letter that is short, to the point, and mail it certified, return receipt requested, to the patient. It can read something like this:

> *Dear Mr. John Doe,*
>
> *I do hope this letter finds you well. With your best medical interest in mind, I will no longer serve as your (insert your field/title here).*
>
> *If you would like to obtain your medical records, please contact the office.*

Here are other practices in the area that may suit your medical needs.
LIST OF LOCAL PRACTICES THAT ARE ACTIVELY ACCEPTING NEW PATIENTS.
Sincerely,
Dr. Doctor

Internal Referral: Another option is to speak with a co-worker to see if he is interested in managing the difficult patient. Sometimes having a male treat another male or a female treat another female, can make the world of difference.

Face-to- Face: If you feel comfortable and the situation presents itself, you can discontinue service with a patient face-to-face. This is the least optimal form of 'firing' a patient, because it puts you and your staff at risk for immediate retaliation. I would not recommend that. Plus, unlike the certified mail, there is no paper trail.

Practitioner Relations

If you have not already, you will encounter doctors, medical assistants, physician assistants, LP nurses, registered nurses, nurse practitioners, et cetera, who are, in short, rude. Unfortunately, the medical field is not exempt from the high school drama that we experienced years ago. First, I encourage you not to be a part of the problem. The practice of medicine is stressful enough, without having to add inter-personal drama to the mix.

When you are dealing with other colleagues, and the situation is not amicable, I do have a few recommendations:

1. Speak with your colleague, personally. Show the respect you would want shown to you. Having someone else relay aggressive or even a constructive criticism message is a sure way to create tension. Plus, you want to be able to relay your point in the manner you intended. Having a third party involved will provide a way for the message to get misconstrued. Remember playing telephone as a kid?

2. Be direct and respectful. I have had colleagues curse at me and point in my face, when they were upset or frustrated. Respect lost. Instead, I would recommend taking a moment to gather your thoughts in an educated way and present them to your peer. Volatile words only add fuel to the flame.

3. When replying to a peer via email, draft a response, but do not send it immediately. Instead, wait until your anger, frustration or rage has subsided. Then, re-read your email

and make changes as needed. Usually, you can find a more mature, professional way to express yourself, when you are not fuming with anger!

4. Try not to discuss your peers with others in the office. It is difficult, and at times unavoidable. Still, you want to maintain as much professionalism as possible. Also, when others are discussing colleagues and co-workers, try not to add to the conversation with your experiences. Like I said, it is not always easy, but if you make it a habit, soon you will find that people stop coming to you with office gossip.

Most of the times, you will be fortunate to work with amazing practitioners who are eager, capable and willing to work with you too. Here are a few tips to help you obtain and maintain healthy professional relationships:

1. Always have business cards with you. Yes, people still use business cards! It might seem antiquated, with all the amazing things our smart phones can do, but healthcare providers are always stuffing things in their pockets-

notes and reminders. You want to make sure you get in their pockets!

2. Eat in the doctors' lounge, or in the common eating area in the hospital. Food is a universal language. It is easy to strike up genuine conversations with people over lunch.

3. When you get a consult or see a mutual patient, be sure to correspond with the other practitioner - letter, phone call – if warranted, or even stop by to inform him of the plan. After a while you will become well known among your peers, and hopefully garner more referrals and consults.

4. When you do meet a new practitioner and numbers/contact information are exchanged, instead of having them save your number under your name, have them save it under your specialty or medical focus. For instance, as a podiatrist, I would have them save it primarily under 'foot doctor', rather than Dr. Josey. Chances are, when they are in need of a podiatrist, they will remember that they met a foot doctor vs Dr. Josey.

Time Saving Tips

Throughout this book I have shared some ways to help expedite your patient encounters without offending your patient or mitigating your patient's experience. Here are a few tips for quick reference.

1. Over time you will realize that there are consistent diagnoses and problems that you will manage. Formulate your treatment plan and protocol for such common diagnoses. That will decrease the time you have to spend trying to formulate a plan 'off the cuff'.

2. Add value without adding time to your patient's visit by making the encounter personalized. Talk about more than just medicine. People equate interest in *them* with *quality* of care.

3. Take control of the length of the visit by redirecting the conversation through questions. Long-winded patients can be pleasant but time consuming. Asking questions is an effective way to regain control and thus allow you to end the visit on your terms.

4. Often times you will have patients with many questions, though the questions are not completely formulated in their minds. This can

make for long pauses and confusion on the patients' part and your part. To help save time tell such patients to write their questions and concerns down and bring them back to the next appointment. Let them know that you want to properly and completely address their concerns. If you have a HIPAA (Health Insurance Portability and Accountability Act) compliant patient communication portal, you can always encourage your patients to communicate with you that way also. Be creative as well as effective when managing your valuable time.

5. Careful patient scheduling is vital to time management and efficient patient visits. Of course you will have to see what works best for you and your staff. I like to have my new patients scheduled in the morning with return patients scattered throughout. Then end the morning with another new patient. The afternoon schedule starts with new patients and ends with return patients. By having a specific format for scheduling patients the flow of your office is steady. Be sure to factor in walk-in patients as well as minor procedure time slots, if appropriate. Some healthcare providers prefer to have specific days blocked

for certain procedures or certain treatments such as injections or palliative care. It is entirely up to you, but I encourage you to have a specific order to your schedule.

6. Each employee and staff member should have complete knowledge of his expected tasks for patient care. If you or your team is uncertain of job descriptions then there will be excessive time spent wondering who is responsible for various tasks. Not to mention that time will be spent repeating requests/orders over and over, as the task responsibility gets passed from person to person. Having multiple parties in the chain of communication gives way to misunderstandings and errors.

7. Your body language is also a great way to politely convey messages to your patient. I have found that there are a few direct and tactful ways to non-verbally indicate that the visit time has ended.

- Standing up from a seated position and heading to the door
- Gathering papers, pens and other charting and heading to the door
- Removing gloves and washing hands/using alcohol based sanitizer

- Casually placing hands in pocket with a smile
- Offering hand for handshake with a smile

8. Frankly stating that the visit is ended, when done correctly, not only helps you manage the length of the visit, but doing so will help direct the patient in the next step. 'Alright Mr. Smith, we are all done here. Be sure to check out at the front desk and schedule your two week follow up appointment.' That statement achieves two goals – the patient understands that the visit is over and he understands that he must follow up in two weeks.

I hope you have found this book helpful. There are so many ways to connect with your patients and staff. I urge you to personalize the tips and ideas presented to fit you and your team! Remember, it takes months to get a new patient, but only seconds to lose one.

Though you are in the medical field, you are also in customer service and sales. Everyone is his own sales representative. Be sure that you are representing the company of YOU, Inc. well.

Staff is the first impression your patient has of the practice. Treat your staff and co-workers well. Happy people are productive people.

I WILL EITHER SEE YOU AT THE TOP OR FROM THE TOP…YOU DECIDE!©

~Dr. S. Simone Josey

Connecting with Dr. Simone Josey:

Online: www.esteemspeaking.weebly.com

Email: esteem.speaking@gmail.com

Mail Correspondence:
Attn: Darlene Smith, Esq.
8715 Apple Blossom Lane
West Chester, OH 45069

Facebook: Dr. Simone Says (Public Figure Page)

Instagram: drsimonesays

Twitter: @drsimonesays

YouTube: DrSimoneSays